PENGUIN BOOKS

ON EATING

Susie Orbach is a psychotherapist. Her books include *Fat is a Feminist Issue* (1978), *Hunger Strike* (Penguin, 1986), *What's Really Going on Here* (1994), *Towards Emotional Literacy* (1999) and *The Impossibility of Sex* (Allen Lane/Penguin Press, 1999). With Luise Eichenbaum she has written *Understanding Women: A Feminist Psychoanalytic Account* (Penguin, 1982), *What Do Women Want: Exploding the Myth of Dependency* (1983) and *Between Women* (1988). She is a Visiting Professor at the London School of Economics.

Susie Orbach
On Eating

PENGUIN BOOKS

PENGUIN BOOKS

Published by the Penguin Group
Penguin Books Ltd, 80 Strand, London WC2R ORL, England
Penguin Putnam Inc., 375 Hudson Street, New York, New York 10014, USA
Penguin Books Australia Ltd, 250 Camberwell Road, Camberwell, Victoria 3124, Australia
Penguin Books Canada Ltd, 10 Alcorn Avenue, Toronto, Ontario, Canada M4V 3B2
Penguin Books India (P) Ltd, 11 Community Centre, Panchsheel Park, New Delhi – 110 017, India
Penguin Books (NZ) Ltd, Cnr Rosedale and Airborne Roads, Albany, Auckland, New Zealand
Penguin Books (South Africa) (Pty) Ltd, 24 Sturdee Avenue, Rosebank 2196, South Africa

Penguin Books Ltd, Registered Offices: 80 Strand, London WC2R ORL, England

On the World Wide Web at: www.penguin.com

First published 2002

14

Copyright © Susie Orbach, 2002

Set in 12/16 pt PostScript Scala Sans Italic
Typeset by Rowland Phototypesetting Ltd, Bury St Edmunds, Suffolk
Printed in England by Clays Ltd, St Ives plc

ISBN-13: 978–0–141–00751–9

To Lianna and Lukas

Thank you to Lianna for delightful help with the mocking up of the pages – more than once; to Caradoc King, Joseph Schwartz and Caroline Pick for their enthusiasm; to Margaret Bluman for another hugely enjoyable and productive time of working together; to Ruth Killick, Rosie Glaisher, Nellie Flexner, Jenny Todd, Andrew Barker and the whole Penguin team for their thoughtfulness and energy.

Contents

How to Use This Book 11

The Keys 17
First Key:
   Eat when you are hungry 19
Second Key:
   Eat the food your body is hungry for 25
Third Key:
   Find out why you eat when you aren't hungry 43
Fourth Key:
   Taste every mouthful 61
Fifth Key:
   Stop eating the moment you are full 75

*Eating to satisfy your hunger is the way to eat
   for the rest of your life* 87
*Changing your eating and changing your body
   image* 90
Eating with your hunger is a guide to living 100

Questions and Answers 105

7

Eating is pleasurable.

Eating is delicious.

Eating is sensual.

But for lots of people, it is also anguishing and fraught with difficulties.

This book gives you keys to transform your eating. From eating that hurts or is chaotic into eating that calms and nourishes you.

How to Use This Book

Take this book slowly. Read a few pages at a time and read them as often as you find helpful.

You may absorb the ideas at first reading. Or you may want to go back to particular parts again and again to understand the ideas and put them into practice.

Sometimes just one key or one page will give you the clue you need.

Order the keys in your personal way. Start with what works best for you. No key is more important than any other. They work together, although any particular one might have special meaning for you.

These ideas are simple. But they will also make demands on you. Grappling with the difficulties you come up against will repay you a thousandfold. You will be free of eating worries for the rest of your life.

First things first.

We each have a mechanism – our personal set point – that regulates our body size. It works best when we eat when we are hungry and stop when we are full.

Eat too little and your metabolism slows down. Your hunger increases as your body tries to get you back to the size that is right for you.

Eat too much and your metabolism also slows down. It can't process the excess food effectively.

Eat what's just right for you and your metabolism will be efficient. Your body will be stable and content at its set point.

As well as our personal set point, we each have an inner register that can tell us:

* how to eat
* when to eat
* what to eat
* when to stop eating.

Eating is like other bodily functions – sleeping, peeing, walking, sneezing. Our body sends us signals, which we can respond to.

This book will help you to respond to your body's inner register. It will be your personal guide to eating.

Undoing years of chaotic or unhealthy eating takes time. Learning to eat in a new way, a way that will work for you for the rest of your life, is like an injured person learning to walk or talk again.

It takes practice before it becomes second nature.

Eating well can become that for you if you give it a chance.

Take your problem seriously.

Give it the attention it needs.

This book shows you how to eat with your hunger and stop when you are full. It isn't magic, it may not happen overnight: it takes work. Sometimes a lot of work. But once you've got the knack, it feels magically different from the way you've eaten before.

Don't expect miracles. Follow the keys. In time you will notice that your eating is relaxed and easy. Better than a miracle.

Eating this way means:

*   *an end to diets*
*   *an end to binges*

*   *an end to special schemes to control your food*
*   *an end to denying yourself the food you would really like to be eating.*

The Keys

Five keys will help you eat in a new way and enable you to be the size that is right for you.

With these keys you will always have the resources to transform your eating if it feels out of control.

Return to them whenever you feel the need. They will provide you with immediate solutions.

These keys give you the way to trust yourself around food, even if you have never been able to do so before.

If you follow them, they are foolproof.

No diet, no doctor, no trainer, no scheme can know better than you what suits your body.

These five keys are always there for you to go to if you get into difficulties or forget them. They don't change.

* They give instant relief to troubled eating.
* You don't have to wait until next Monday.
* You can start right now.
* Today.

First Key

Eat when you are hungry.

Eat when you are hungry.

Don't wait until you are very very hungry or starving.

If you have no idea when you are hungry, do not eat.

It means you aren't hungry.

You may have messed about so much with your hunger signals that you have to learn about them again.

In either case, do not eat unless you feel hunger pangs.

Learning to discover your hunger signals can take a bit of practice and a lot of attention.

Your aim is to get your hunger signals to work as clearly as the one that tells you when to pee. This signal tells you that:

* sometimes you need to pee a lot
* sometimes there's just a trickle.

Whatever the volume, your body tells you and you respond.

So too with hunger. Your hunger signals can tell you that:

* sometimes your body will want to eat a lot
* sometimes your body wants just a little.

It isn't always the same and there may not be a pattern. But whatever the amount your body needs, it can give you the right signal.

Hints

The hunger mechanism will be there if you let it emerge and then treat it right when it does.

* *Some people feel hunger in their belly.*
* *Some in their chest.*
* *Some in their throat.*

As long as you don't interrupt the process by eating before you feel it, you'll get your personal signal, the one that lets you know it is time for you to eat.

If you are not used to recognizing your hunger, don't despair. There are reasons.

Perhaps you don't know when you are hungry because:

* you eat before you get hungry

* you eat because everyone else is eating

* you eat because you are miserable, weepy, angry

* you eat because you are happy

* you eat because you passed a bakery with wonderful smells

* you eat because it's mealtime

* you eat because your mother told you to

* you eat because you feel fat and hopeless

* you eat because you are bored

* you eat the food your child left over.

Sometimes we can be afraid to feel our hunger. The very sensation frightens us and so we eat in advance of it or try to ignore it.

That can happen because as children:

* we didn't have enough food
* we had to clear our plates whether we wanted to or not
* we sensed our mother's disapproval if we said we weren't hungry
* eating was the shared family activity.

This book will help you find out the personal emotional reasons why hunger is something you might be reluctant to feel.

Knowing those reasons clears the way for you to use your hunger to guide your eating.

Second Key

Eat the food your body
is hungry for.

Eat the food your body is hungry for.

Eat what you really desire.

No rules, no regulations.

No bad foods, no good foods.

Most of us think chocolate, cakes, cream, crisps and sweets are bad and sinful.

There was a time when bread, rice, potatoes and pasta were thought of as bad and meat as good.

Now we think that vegetables, bread, grain, pasta, low-fat foods, fish and fruit are good.

What is thought to be healthy is as much to do with nutrition fashion as it is to do with science or truth.

It is easy to get stressed about the wholesomeness of our foods. So many foods today are made with excessive chemicals and some taste as though they've been grown in a lab.

Distinguish between foods that can harm you because they are made up of chemicals and flavourings and aren't really food, and foods you designate bad, such as ice cream, puddings and french fries, because they are highly calorific or associated with treats.

We can be tempted to call whole categories of foods bad as a way to put them off limits. We cordon them off and avoid them when what is really going on is that we don't know how to handle them.

When we call a food 'bad', we exclude it from what we allow ourselves to eat.

Or we attach conditions to when we can and can't (usually can't) eat it.

But these strategies don't work because a 'bad' food inevitably becomes extra tempting.

We try to resist the food but end up eating our way through the good foods we aren't hungry for to get to those foods we've decided are off limits or bad.

As we eat the 'bad' food, we attack ourselves for doing so.

Denying yourself particular foods is a recipe for bingeing and hurting.

If you banish or forbid yourself a particular food, you crave endless amounts of it. When you do let go and eat it, you start to binge.

You promise yourself you won't eat it again. This is the last time you'll indulge, lose control, let yourself go. So, inevitably, you cram the last of it into you now.

Then you feel guilty. You are unable to enjoy or savour this food that you've made forbidden or bad.

This is a terrible shame. A double punishment.

When you eat *what* you really want *and the
food fits your hunger and satisfies you, it is
good.*

Chocolate cake eaten because you are hungry
for it in your mouth and in your stomach can be
relished. It answers that hunger and you won't
need anything else until you are hungry again.

Contrast that with eating it guiltily after you
have ploughed through a meal in order to get it.

Which tastes better?

Which is more satisfying?

If you discover there are certain foods you are really afraid to eat because they send you on a binge, allow yourself to get to know them all over again.

Have that food as a meal the next time you are hungry for it.

Taste it.

Really concentrate on it.

Get the most out of it.

Let it fill you up with its luxurious flavour and texture.

If it is as wonderful as you imagined it to be, treat it as such. Let it be worthy of your attention, not just something that has to be sneaked into your mouth when you aren't noticing because you aren't meant to be having it in the first place.

A wonderfully pleasurable food deserves respect, not just swallowing or getting it over and done with as though there was something wrong with you for wanting it or having it.

Work out the rules that exist in your head about foods.

* What are your good foods?
* What are your bad foods?
* When do you allow yourself to eat these foods?

You might think meals are all right.
Or perhaps eating before 6.00 p.m.
Or that anything low fat or vegetable is harmless.

Almost everyone has sets of competing rules in their heads about food, usually based on rather flimsy information.

Take a look at your rules and see how some of them contradict one another.

Realize too that they haven't worked.
That's obvious.
Let them go.
Instead, eat what you are hungry for.

To find out what you **are** hungry for imagine yourself eating the food you want.

It might be something you don't usually let yourself have.

It might be foods from your childhood.

It might be foods from before you started dieting.

It might be foods that you eat now but pretend to yourself you aren't really eating.

It might be foods you have rarely tasted because you have decided that they are off limits.

Whatever it is, imagine this food.

Take a minute to think about:

* the taste of it
* the smell of it
* the feel of it in your mouth.

If you are still hungry for it, eat it. See how it tastes and whether you enjoy it as much as you hoped you would.

If you find you no longer want that specific food, imagine eating, smelling, tasting something else.

If you are still hungry for this food, eat it. See how it tastes and whether you enjoy it as much as you hoped you would.

If no food you imagine seems to match your hunger, perhaps you aren't hungry for food at all.

Maybe what you are really hungry for is:

* a hug
* a weep
* a sleep
* a break
* a boyfriend
* a chat with your friend.

Give yourself time to discover what you are really hungry for.

Hints

If you are so unused to allowing yourself to eat what you want because you've been involved in limiting your foods in different ways, discover what foods interest you now by taking a trip around your favourite deli, supermarket, restaurant, café or the kitchen of your childhood.

If that feels too dangerous imagine doing it in your head first. Knowing that you are safe, that the food won't leap at you, look at the huge variety of foods; their colours, their textures, their smells.

When you have got used to this idea in your imagination, do it in real life.

Notice which foods beckon to you.

Imagine you can have anything and everything there, **for ever**.

Whenever you eat something it will be replaced.

There is no such thing as clearing your plate or finishing the packet of biscuits; only endless gorgeous food.

Make a list of your favourite foods and imagine yourself eating them.

Discover which circumstances let you eat perfectly with your hunger.

Is it cooking for yourself?

Is it being cooked for by a friend?

Is it eating in a restaurant?

Is it eating a take-out?

Is it eating alone?

Use this information to help you eat what your body is hungry for.

*Choose **only** foods you love.*

Choose foods that sit well within your body.

Choose foods that satisfy you.

Third Key

Find out why you eat when you aren't hungry.

Find out why you eat when you aren't hungry.

Address the reasons directly.

Food can only satisfy stomach hunger.

It cannot make other hungers go away.

It can only postpone them or temporarily cover them up.

If you are lonely and you eat, you will have given yourself a reason why you are lonely – 'I'm too fat and therefore I am lonely.'

You won't have addressed your loneliness; rather you will have taken yourself a step away from solving it.

You will also – without meaning to – have given yourself an extra problem: a food problem.

If you eat when you need to cry, your tears will always be there waiting to be shed.

If you eat when you are angry, you are swallowing a feeling that needs to come out.

If you eat when you are feeling lost, you may feel more lost.

Allow yourself the idea that you might not be hungry for food at all.

Your hunger might be emotional.

Food cannot satisfy other kinds of hungers.

It can quiet them momentarily but, when you are finished eating, they are still there.

The food you eat to temporarily quell your emotions can't actually do that. It is you – not the food – who is quieting the uneasy emotion.

You can't always respond to your emotional hungers.

You won't always know what is troubling you.

You may not have the words.

You may be ashamed of certain feelings.

But that doesn't mean that covering them up with food is a solution.

If you are eating when you aren't hungry, stop and ask yourself what you are hungry for.

If you can't come up with an answer, and don't know what exactly you need at that time, don't despair.

This is not a reason to eat. It is a reason to be pleased with yourself for not eating and not adding to your original problem.

If you can't work out what you are feeling and what would be satisfying, try feeling regret about not knowing the answer.

Recognizing you don't know will calm and soothe you more successfully than eating when you are not physically hungry for food.

Hints

If you can't fathom your emotional hungers, or
are too afraid of them, don't worry.

Here are some things you can do to give yourself
the space to find out:

* write some sentences asking yourself what
  you are hungry for
* take a bath
* cuddle up and read a book
* take a walk
* phone a friend
* draw a picture.

There may be something that is troubling you
that you can't quite put your finger on.

Even though you don't yet know what it is,
you've stopped yourself falling into the food and
adding to your problems.

Perhaps you have uncomfortable feelings that make no sense to you. You feel unhappy or angry. You don't know or understand why. You wish the feelings would just go away. You push them away but they come back.

If you can acknowledge these uncomfortable feelings, they won't have to plague you.

Perhaps you are feeling excited or delighted. Perhaps you are feeling calm. Each person has feelings they are unused to coping with, even pleasurable ones.

We expect positive feelings to be easy, but they too can be troublesome.

Feelings are very similar to food. If you pay attention to the feeling, if you allow yourself to experience it, it will fill you up. Sometimes you will be filled up with sadness, sometimes with anger, sometimes with joy. When your personal feelings fill you up, you will feel better even if the feelings are sad ones.

Being able to put names to the emotions that lie behind your wish to eat when you aren't physically hungry is the most nourishing food you can give yourself.

Notice the emotions you are most comfortable with.
Write them down.

Notice the emotions that make you uneasy.
Write those down too.

For example, if you feel nervous or reluctant to acknowledge your anger, think about why.

Did you come from an angry or violent home?

Or were you never allowed to express anger when you were growing up?

Think about the personal reasons why you regard anger in the way that you do.

Remember anger is just a feeling like any other. You may not be easy with it but you can learn to accept it. You don't always have to show it just because you feel it.

And what about the feelings close to anger?

Can you accept feelings of helplessness?

Can you allow yourself to feel sad?

Can you recognize rage in yourself?

Is disappointment a feeling you know?

Is it difficult to admit to feeling depressed?

These emotions can be hard to accept.

But you don't have to do anything with them, just experience them privately, for yourself.

Even if you are uneasy with feelings of this sort, naming them and experiencing them lets you know what they are like.

Instead of keeping them at a distance, where they can threaten you, feeling them lessens their menace. They may be uncomfortable or disconcerting, they may make you feel sad or in pain, but as you get to know them your confidence in handling them will make you less afraid of yourself.

Knowing them in this way will help you with your eating.

When you want to eat but you know you aren't really hungry, you can ask yourself:

Am I angry?

Am I sad?

Am I feeling helpless?

Am I in a rage?

Am I disappointed?

Am I depressed?

Am I excited?

Often there will be nothing you need to do about your private feelings.

* They don't have to be acted on.
* They don't have to be run away from.
* They don't have to be turned into something else.
* They don't have to be taken out on somebody else.

They are just part of what makes you human in your own unique way.

You might not be able to work out the emotional reasons why you might want to eat when you aren't physically hungry. That's OK.

You are looking for clues to help you find the feelings and activities that will satisfy your real emotional hungers. That way you can keep food and eating for when you are physically hungry.

Fourth Key

Taste every mouthful.

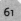

Taste every mouthful.

Taste.
Notice.
Enjoy every bite.

It doesn't matter how much you paid for it.
It doesn't matter how long it took to prepare.

If you aren't tasting the food 100 per cent
you don't need it
and it is doing you no good.

Don't waste even one mouthful of pleasure.

Stop eating the moment you stop savouring the food or the moment your mind wanders away from the sensation of the food.

If you've been eating chaotically, every eating experience from now on is a chance to change that.

Each time you eat when you are hungry and you eat **exactly** what is right for your body you are building confidence.

You are learning that you can feed yourself and look after yourself too.

Don't cheat yourself of the deep pleasure of eating well.

Pay attention to what your stomach really wants.

Notice which foods really please and satisfy you.

Notice the foods that leave you feeling uncomfortable.

Observe which foods are so moreish you feel you can't stop eating them.

When this happens it means that your taste buds rather than your hunger have taken over.

If sugary things make you crave more sugar so that you feel you really can't stop, eat the sweet food first rather than last.

If you are eating a meal this might mean starting with dessert and having other foods as a second course.

Following dessert with fish or pasta or noodles will quell the urge for the sweet taste.

You won't be depriving yourself.

The sweet food doesn't become a bad food that has to be avoided.

You can have the sweet thing you find delicious in a way that feels safe.

See how the foods you eat sit in your body.

Do they make you feel good?

Do they give you energy?

Do they make you feel drowsy?

Do they make you feel sick?

Notice which foods leave you with contented feelings after eating them.

Notice which foods taste good in your mouth but feel awful when you are digesting them.

Certain foods may disagree with you. This could be any kind of food. Our bodies are very personal. Sometimes the way we respond to a specific food depends on when we eat it. We can digest it better in the morning than at night. Sometimes whole groups of foods – meat, nuts, dairy – don't agree with us. Each of us needs to find out how specific foods affect us.

Some foods may:

* bring you out in hives
* make you feel bloated
* make you feel hyper.

Be wise and avoid them.

It might make you feel a little sad that your body rebels when you eat certain foods, but you need to respect your body's reactions and feel the regret that certain foods you like the taste of aren't for you.

There are plenty of delicious foods that will nourish you without producing a negative reaction in your body.

If you crave endless amounts of a particular food even when you realize your hunger has been satisfied, this particular food probably doesn't agree with you.

Perhaps you are responding to the sugar or salt in the food and the chemical receptors in your brain crave more of those flavourings. Your salt and sugar receptors are working overtime and will never be satisfied. Once you have gone beyond a small portion there actually is no right amount. It becomes hard for you to stop because you are not responding to hunger but to a craving that has been induced by the salt or sugar.

This doesn't mean never eating sugar or salt. It does mean being aware of their effect on you and eating them alongside or backed up by other foods that neutralize the craving effects of the sugar and salt.

Hints

If you are in danger of eating everything that's put before you, try to leave a mouthful of every type of food on your plate.

When someone else is deciding how much shall go on your plate, or even when you have served yourself, leaving a little of each food begins to put you in control of your food.

This will help you to discover the right amount for you.

If certain foods worry you, if sweets, bread or bananas scare you, try having enough of the particular food around you so that you can never eat it all.

If you think you could binge on:

* 3 chocolate bars
* a packet of biscuits
* a pot of chocolate mousse

keep 8 or 10 times as many of them in the house.

This may sound a strange thing to try but this is how to change the mystique associated with these foods. If you have plenty of them around, more than you could possibly eat in one go, you will start to see them just as foods, foods you enjoy, foods that are staples to have when you are hungry for them.

Gradually, you will experience yourself as able to select these once bingey foods in a positive way. You won't rush to finish them or banish them because they are sitting there challenging or threatening you.

When you do make the choice to eat those foods you will fully savour and enjoy them.

To help you if you lose attention while you eat, carry a small notebook and pen with you.

* If you notice yourself eating more than you are hungry for
* if you are eating without noticing
* if your fork or spoon is going to your mouth automatically
* if it ceases to matter what you are eating

stop:
Take out your notebook and jot down your thoughts.

Notice the thoughts that have turned your focus away from your eating.

Are they negative, disconcerting or frightening thoughts?

Are they exciting or pleasurable thoughts?

Turn your attention to them. They are more important than eating right now.

If you are eating with others when this happens, you can still stop eating and quietly go inside yourself to register the thoughts that are claiming your attention.

If you can't write them down or think about them at the time, remind yourself to do so later. They matter. They can help you understand why you eat when you are not hungry.

Knowing yourself more fully will allow you to interrupt the habit of eating without awareness.

Fifth Key

*Stop eating the
moment you are full.*

Stop eating the moment you are full.

Don't blunt that feeling. It is truly great.

It draws a line between eating and not eating.

* Start to eat when you are genuinely hungry.

* Pay attention while you are eating.

* Stop as soon as you are full.

It is much easier to notice when you are full if you stay alert while you are eating.

If you savour every mouthful, you won't feel cheated. The sense of fullness won't come too soon and you will be ready to stop eating.

Your body will send you a message that it is satisfied.

If you don't concentrate while you eat, your body may be telling you it's full but you may still be wanting more taste sensations in your mouth.

You will be tempted to override the feeling of fullness because you have missed part of the enjoyment of the food.

You can't afford to do that if you are trying to get your hunger and satisfaction signals to work accurately.

If you start to eat when you aren't hungry, there was never a biological reason to start and there won't be a biological signal to help you stop.

If you discover that you aren't hungry for very much, don't worry. You will be hungry again soon.

Promise yourself that you will eat what you want the next time you are hungry.

Do not use a small hunger to see how long you can go without food.

Eat when your body lets you know that you are hungry.

If you eat when you are hungry your body rewards you:

* It uses your food properly.
* Your metabolism works correctly.
* You digest well what you put in your body.
* You will know when you need to eat again.

If you know you will be away from a source of food, discover and think about the foods you can take with you that will really please you.

Carry a small selection with you.

Hints

Eating when you are hungry and paying attention to the pleasure of the foods lets you know when you are full.

If you have no idea how to sense that you are full, take the following steps to learn:

* Eat just what you estimate might be the right amount and then take a pause.
* Get away from where you are eating.
* Involve yourself in another activity.
* Check back on your stomach in fifteen minutes.
* If you are still hungry, see what it is you are hungry for now, and then pay close attention while you eat it.

If you are eating with others you may want to be private about what you are doing.

Invent a phone call you have to make or excuse yourself and go to the toilet with a book for a few minutes.

Give yourself a chance to be immersed in another activity and see whether your hunger is still calling you.

If you find you are still hungry, choose the foods that will satisfy that hunger.

If you realize that you are **not** hungry but you know this is one of those times when you want to go on eating, be even more selective.

See if you can judge what kind of food will do the trick.
Do you want something:

* hard to bite?
* hot and liquidy?
* sweet and sticky?
* smooth and bland?
* sour and savoury?

Don't just eat.

Choose.

Choosing helps you to get the right food for your mood.
Choosing makes you feel less insatiable and out of control.
Choosing short-circuits a binge.

Eating to Satisfy Your Hunger is the Way to Eat for the Rest of Your Life

These five keys:

* eating when you are hungry
* eating the food you are hungry for
* finding out why you want to eat when you aren't hungry
* tasting every mouthful
* stopping when you are full

will hold you steady and give you a new, reliable and nourishing way to eat.

They will give you sensual satisfaction.

They will allow your body to process what you eat properly.

When we eat too little our body acts as if there were a food shortage:

* it adjusts to the reduced rations and conserves the food
* our body's metabolism slows down.

When we eat more than our body needs:

* our metabolism also slows down
* it cannot process the excess.

When we eat just what our body needs, our metabolism speeds up and works properly.

If you feel that your body is stuck and your metabolism is flat, build up to 40 minutes of continuous physical exercise, such as:

* *walking*
* *jogging*
* *swimming*
* *weight training*
* *dancing*

three times a week.

This kind of activity kick-starts a sluggish system. Exercise can also give you a different and positive experience of your body.

Changing Your Eating and Changing Your Body Image

There are many reasons why people eat more than their bodies need.

Some of these have to do with the ideas we have about our body size.

Most of us believe that we will be happier if we are thinner. That message constantly bombards us. So we try to change our bodies to be thinner.

That's usually how we get into trouble with food in the first place. We ignore our stomach hunger and try to know better than our bodies how much and when we should be eating.

Then our minds and our mouths rebel. We get bigger rather than smaller. If we are dieting we only stay smaller through excessive rules and regulations. But dieting actually makes you fatter because it interrupts your body's natural signals and slows down your metabolism.

When you do start to eat when you are hungry and stop when you are full after years of being on one scheme or another, you will most likely go down a size or several sizes.

Unless you have been eating drastically less than your body needs for years, your weight should stabilize at its natural set point, which will be lower than what you've achieved through dieting and bingeing.

Think about how you would feel about being thinner.

Many people imagine they would automatically feel more confident, sexier and happier if they were thinner. They feel certain they would cope with their problems better.

In fact, they can feel less sure of themselves. They may not cope better or be happier, more confident and sexier.

They may think they have to or want to act sexier and more confident but it isn't really them and so they can't sustain it.

They often gain weight again because they don't know how to handle the expectations they have for themselves.

Knowing your personal expectations can help you avoid this trap.

If you think you want to be thinner, in what ways will you expect different things of yourself?

Are there things you don't do now that you would do if you were thinner?

Make a list of what you imagine would be different.

Are there things you are doing now that you imagine you would not be doing if you were thinner?

93

Ask yourself in which ways, apart from your size, you are expecting yourself to change?

Are these expectations realistic?

When you imagine yourself thinner is it you you see or someone else?

You need to get used to a new body image if you want to be smaller or thinner.

Accustom yourself to seeing yourself as the thinner you.

Walk, sit, move as though you were the size you want to be. Wear your clothes. See yourself in your home. See yourself at work. Inhabit that new body.

If you can't imagine yourself thinner in your milieu, then it might be your life you are wanting to change, not your size. Size only changes size. It doesn't change your life.

If you can see yourself thinner doing everyday things, then it won't be such a surprise or shock when you get there.

If you are *imagining yourself as a different person when you become thinner, and want to develop those aspects of yourself, try to do so now.*

Experiment with those 'new' parts of yourself.

If you imagine you would be more confident or sexier, try to access that part of you now.

It really doesn't have to do with size.

Act as you would if you were your ideal size.

Don't miss out on your life until you think you are the 'right' size.

Practise and develop those neglected parts of you that you've always put on hold until you become thin.

When you achieve the size you want to be, you won't be a stranger to yourself.

If you think you might be:

* more outgoing
* sexier
* funnier
* quieter
* cleverer
* more desirable
* flirtatious
* hard-working
* studious
* responsible
* and so on

try enhancing those wanted aspects of you now.

They are not to do with size.

Get to know the parts of you waiting in the wings.

Make them part of who you are now, whatever your size.

They won't disappear when your body image changes.

Are there advantages to being the size you are now? Your immediate response may well be 'no', but slow yourself down and consider the question again: are there any advantages in being your current size?

Might you lose them if you were thinner?

Perhaps you worry that:

* more will be expected of you
* you will feel too visible
* people will see you differently.

Make a list of your personal worries about being thinner.

What positive ideas have you put on to the size you are now?

You do not need to give up any of the things that are important to you, whatever your size.

What negative ideas have you attached to your size now?

Be aware that negative thoughts about your size will not necessarily disappear if you change physically. You may have attached them to size but they may be about other things.

The lovely things about you, your vulnerabilities and your strengths, will find a space within you at all sizes.

Eating with Your Hunger is a Guide to Living

Eating what you want when you are hungry and stopping when you are full is a foundation for dealing with your other needs and desires.

If you know when you are hungry for food and you know how to satisfy stomach hunger, then you have a guide for dealing with your other appetites.

You will be able to be more welcoming and less afraid of your needs in general.

You will have learnt that you can cope with different kinds of wantings.

You'll be able to observe your desires. You won't have to eat over them. You won't have to hurry to fulfil them. You will be able to wait to see what to do with that particular need.

You will be able to recognize that powerful or insistent desires that you've been wary of, or not known how to address, can be lived with.

* *They don't have to be eaten away.*
* *They don't have to be denied.*
* *They don't have to be responded to immediately.*

It takes time to get used to the idea that you won't instantly know what to do with a particular need.

Slowly you will see that you can acknowledge your desires and longings to yourself.

You will get used to letting them sit inside of you until you discover the right way to handle them.

Knowing that you can handle your food and your other needs a little at a time is very reassuring.

It cuts into the idea that you are insatiable and can never be satisfied.

You will be able to enjoy and digest not just your food, but recognize and digest your feelings too.

As you take in the right amount of food for you, so you will be learning about how to cope with the emotional atmosphere around you.

You won't be able to stop dramas or bad things happening – that's part of living – but you will have new energy and tools to deal with your emotional responses.

You won't be eating your problems away. You will be looking at them and finding new ways to deal with them. You will be feeding your stomach when it is hungry and responding to your emotional states directly.

You will be dealing with life problems and life solutions, not life problems turned into food problems and phoney food solutions.

Questions and Answers

What do I do if I am going out for supper and I am not hungry? I was hungry at 5 p.m. and ate then. I don't want to appear rude.

Next time, try eating a small amount of something really satisfying at 5.00 p.m. Remind yourself you will have the option to eat again in a few hours. Stopping will not be a deprivation but a way for you to also enjoy the food later.

My family wants me to eat with them and to eat what they are eating but it doesn't suit me.

This can be a tricky transition. Family meals have significance for all of us. Changing the routine can upset people even if they have accommodated to various diets and eating schemes before. Explaining why it's important to you can help, as can sitting with them while they are eating so you don't lose that time together. Another option is to have the meal around your appetite and your favourites so that they eat what you desire.

My boyfriend has booked a special meal for our anniversary but I realize now that I eat with my hunger best when I am on my own. I feel bad because he is paying a lot for it. I feel I'll have to eat it all.

I'm sure your boyfriend wants you to enjoy your meal and sees it as an act of love to eat together. Use it to experiment how to eat exactly what you want when you are out with him. Don't expect 100 per cent perfection first time; see this as a process towards getting your appetite, food and boyfriend harmonized. Most restaurants will be happy to give you first-course-size dishes or two first courses and dessert or make adjustments to their menu. And if you leave food on your plate because you have had enough and they ask, 'Was everything all right?' they are satisfied if you say, 'Delicious, I just couldn't manage more.'

Everyone is eating lunch and then we are going for a long walk. I'm not hungry but won't have a chance to eat later. How do I handle this?

There is nothing wrong with saying that you just don't have the appetite for food now and either making a sandwich to take with you or asking the restaurant to make something up for you to take.

I never want to eat when I fall in love but when I get into the relationship I balloon up.

Infatuation and falling in love are well-known appetite suppressants but what's also going on is that we are filled up with feelings – in this case, especially pleasurable ones. All feelings, if we let them, are capable of filling us up. The hole we sometimes mistakenly call hunger often has to do with being devoid of our feelings, whatever they are.

Of course, when a relationship gets going, we have to face our disappointments with our partners, the fact that they are real people with differences from us, rather than being perfectly tuned-in and adoring us at all times. We also have to realize that sometimes daily intimacy can be difficult and we shy away from it, putting barriers up – including eating – as a way to avoid our own, and our partner's, conflicts about closeness.

Trying to stay with our feelings, whatever they are, is a recipe for not getting muddled about which are issues the relationship needs to address and which are the personal issues. Ballooning up means you've given up focusing on feelings and are focusing on food. You've turned food into the issue rather than what sits between the two of you.

My husband is getting really cross about this new way of eating. He is always trying to tempt me to eat things with him and it is so hard not to. I feel awful refusing him. But I'm losing weight so I don't want to stop doing it.

Perhaps your husband is feeling nervous about your new ease with your food and its impact on your body. Maybe he needs some reassurance on that front.

Try to spend some food times together but explain to him that you eat treats every time you are hungry now.

None of the girls at school have lunch because they are slimming and I would feel really odd eating. I have quite a big appetite.

It's very worrying that girls are skipping meals. I think you have to be the brave one and declare your appetite and be different. Show them how you enjoy your food and the energy it gives you. Perhaps you can even argue with them about their adaptation so that they feel less freaked about eating. Tell them the golden rule: that your body uses the food efficiently when you eat when you are hungry but slows down if you are starving yourself.

Whenever I eat chocolate these days I crave even more of it.

Chocolate does affect some people this way. If you feel afraid of it, make sure that you are eating it only when you really really want it, and when you do have it, make it into a ceremony, don't blank out when you eat it. And think about having something to follow it so the chocolate receptors in your mouth don't keep screaming 'Chocolate!'.

If I eat one salty nut I have to finish the bowl.

It's awful to think that salty nuts should be off limits for you but, if however many you eat you will be craving more because you are going for the salt, you might as well try stopping after a few because the ending is going to be the same whenever you do it.

My gym teacher/trainer says I have to eat according to a set of rules . . .

Yes, trainers often think that a special nutritional programme will do wonders for you without realizing the emotional aspects of eating. They can come up with schemes that help build your muscles or help endurance or lose body fat but these are schemes that depend upon their knowledge of the body, not their knowledge of *your* body. They don't know how many schemes you've tried before and been successful on for short periods of time before reverting to the more chaotic pattern of your eating.

You need to discover your own hungers and what can really sustain you rather than grabbing the latest plan from a trainer or nutritionist who doesn't understand your particular difficulties.

The other thing to be aware of is that many gym teachers and trainers have body-image and food problems of their own. If you listen to the conversations they have among themselves you will hear how familiar their preoccupations are. They try out new schemes themselves because, often, they haven't found a way to eat easily with their own appetites and, although they wouldn't phrase it this way – their language is now in terms of health and fitness – many of them are still looking for solutions to their own eating problems.

Do I have to go to the gym for this to work?

No, you don't have to go to a gym for this to work but having another experience of your body through moving – walking, dancing or sporting – will give you a sense of your body's potential from another perspective and you might find that helpful and even enjoyable.

I have diabetes; how can I use the ideas here?
They scare me.

I have worked with many people who have
diabetes over the years using these five keys
and it has been very successful. Knowing you
have to monitor what your body needs very
precisely and that certain foods interfere with
you being well is simply an extension of the
ideas in this book. Yes, you might have to
recognize that you can't have particular foods
without there being consequences, or you
might discover that there are foods you've
excluded from your diet that you are able to
eat if you back them up with slower-acting
carbohydrates, but this is really all part of
understanding what foods work for you. It
would be foolish and dangerous to mess
about with your blood-sugar levels, and the
five keys are all about enabling you to tune
into your personal needs and respond as
best as you can to them.

Scientists are constantly telling us that certain foods are good for us one minute, and then changing their minds the next. How do we know what to believe?

Yes, it is very tricky trying to keep up with changing nutritional theories, particularly when whatever is new is proclaimed as the truth. Now the US government is back-pedalling from a thirty-year propaganda exercise about low fat to lower cholesterol, as its supposed beneficial impact on heart disease has not been borne out. The thing to do is to notice how different foods affect one individually, eat the ones that make you feel good during and after eating and avoid those that give you only short-term pleasure.

Is fast food really that bad for you?

The important thing to work out is which fast foods agree with you, satisfy you and fill you up, and which don't.

When I am stressed – I can't eat. I have no appetite and I physically feel sick when I try to eat. This was the case at Christmas when I was moving house and splitting up with my boyfriend. Doing yoga helped but only on the days on which I did yoga.

It sounds like your body goes into a shut-down mode when you are sad or stressed and you don't feel terribly alive. The difficulty is that if you can't eat then you lose even more energy and that can make you feel weak and sick. The yoga probably gave you a different and more alive sense of your body, even though your heart was heavy, and made a physical demand on your body, which then restored your appetite. Perhaps recognizing your upset but doing something physical, such as walking, when you are blue would be a way to stimulate your appetite so that the vulnerability you feel emotionally doesn't have to be taken out on your body.

Why do I keep eating when I'm full?

Partly it is because you are used to it and lose awareness while you are eating. But it is probably the case that you have some kind of emotional investment in doing so. A way to find out what that is is to risk not eating beyond full. Keep a notebook with you and write down what you experience. You will most likely come up with a few reasons why you've found it useful to eat beyond your hunger in the past, which, once you've identified, can help you stop when you are full now.

Is it better to 'graze' all day, or have three square meals?

Neither is better. Some people are satisfied by small amounts often and others need the feeling of a meal to be content. And it isn't always the same. There is no ultimate truth about this, just the noticing of what works best in your body at different times.

Why, when I know how much rubbish they contain, do I still crave burgers?

If you associate particular foods as a treat then you will crave them until you have allowed yourself to have them as part of your regular pattern of eating. If you make them a less special food then you will be able to have them without it setting up a craving.

Why do I crave greasy food after a big night out?

Your body is probably exhausted. The greasy food soaks up the alcohol from the night before and boosts you while you are fatigued.

Why does your body seem to crave sugar around the time of your period and sometimes in the afternoon? Can fruit really satisfy this sort of craving?

Often women experience a drop in energy and feel that sugar or carbohydrates help. Another solution is to slow down when you have less umph but that isn't always possible. And if fruit does it for you, great!

Are you heavier at different times of the month?

Yes, I think we have about a 3-kilo fluctuation or so. Everyone does and we usually have a slightly higher weight in winter than summer to protect us if we get colds and lose our appetites. That's why scales can be a ridiculous thing to measure oneself by. They don't ever tell you more than you can know by how your clothes fit or how your body looks.

What foods can help me get started in the mornings?

There are lots of different theories about what gets you going so you'll have to find the foods that are right for you by experimenting. Don't be afraid to try foods you've never considered before. They might do the trick. If you have no idea, imagine yourself ready to eat with an appetite, ready for the day: close your eyes and cast your mind over various food possibilities. Imagine yourself eating and drinking whatever combinations until you hit on something that feels absolutely perfect. It won't always be the same every day but using your imagination in advance to expand the range of what you choose is a good place to start.

Do you believe in listening to your body telling you what it needs? An obvious example is during pregnancy, when those messages are difficult to ignore. What should I do when my body seems to crave caffeine, sugar or carbohydrate?

Any time you have repetitive cravings outside of pregnancy, as opposed to desires for foods, it probably means that you are hooked on that food. It is a chemical push towards the food rather than the expression of your hunger. The spontaneous response to hungers in pregnancy is what you are aiming for all the time.

I consider myself to be too thin but whatever I eat or however much I eat I cannot put on weight. Why?

That's just the way your body processes food. You've got a fast-acting metabolism.

Why is it so hard not to raid the fridge when I get home from work?

Perhaps you go to the fridge much as you might have when you used to come home from school: symbolically getting some feeding from your mum as you did when you were younger. Or perhaps it could be a way of touching base with yourself and the things you now provide for yourself. The fact that you have noticed this habit gives you a chance to make a choice. Do you want to be doing this or would you rather find a less frantic transition point for yourself and leave eating for when you are hungry and can relish it?

Exhaustion (especially coupled with anxiety or stress) seems to provoke an instinctive desire for sugar and thus lead to over-consumption of sweet things. Is this true?

No, I think it's more that there is a tendency to try to get energy quickly when you are exhausted and there is nothing faster than sugar. Taking sugar in a more complex form along with other food groups (like in a smoothie or a granola bar) or eating sugar backed up by something more slow acting will sustain you for longer. Of course, sleep is what you are really craving when you are exhausted, not food at all.

How can I stop snacking in the afternoon?
I always get really hungry about 4–5 p.m. and
don't eat dinner till 7–8 p.m., depending on
when I get home, so I pig out on bread, etc.

Don't stop snacking. Have something that will really satisfy your hunger at 4.00ish. Your body wants food then so find foods that you can have then that will nourish you. You won't be ravenous when you get home and you can decide what you are hungry for without being under the pressure of starvation.

Do you believe that each individual has their own intolerances to certain food types, and that there are few 'blanket rules' to eating/diet?

I can see the attraction of various schemes to manage appetite, to boost health, and so on but I have also seen so many of these 'diets' discredited that I have come to believe that their value for most people is in helping them to regulate their food. The schemes don't actually address issues of appetite and how to deal with what works for your body and how to separate out the emotional issues involved in eating when you aren't hungry.

Why have I suddenly begun to pile on the weight? I eat the same diet, exercise in the same way, work in the same way. Is it because I am in my mid-40s?

'Fraid so. Our metabolism does slow down as we age and provides us with more bulk, so we usually go up a size or two. If it really troubles you, you can try to increase your metabolic rate by doing more exercise or be even more precise about paying attention to every single mouthful.

I'm vegetarian and sometimes find myself getting tired and headachy. My doctor told me this is because of iron deficiency. What can I do to boost my iron (and energy) levels without having to eat meat?

Dried apricots, currants, baked potatoes with their skins, whole grain, dried beans, dark green leafy vegetables, almonds, peanuts, beets, turnips, all are rich in iron. If you eat a fresh orange or increase your intake of vitamin C it might help you absorb the iron more effectively.

I eat a healthy diet of fresh veg and pasta and try not to eat sweets or desserts but I still feel lethargic mid-afternoon and particularly weak after cycling home from work. What am I doing wrong?

You aren't responding to those afternoon signals about hunger! Try having a sustaining snack just before you start to fade, that way you'll be able to make choices about what to eat when you get home rather than having to cram things into a depleted body.

Asking myself all these questions about my feelings seems to be changing me so much. It's not that I don't like it, but I am different now.

Getting to know yourself and reflecting on your past experiences with food, and thinking and feeling what is right for you now, does involve change and that might feel both exciting as well as a bit unfamiliar and scary even. It can be strange and even hard to give up an image of yourself as someone who is out of control around food when that is no longer happening and to adjust to who you are becoming, but it can also be reassuring to know that you have put into place changes you really wanted.

If dieting is the answer, what's the question?

And remember: scales are for fish not people.